"She'll never live." Those were the first words my mother heard from her nurse after I was delivered. "Your daughter is blue, weighs only 3 pounds, and has some kind of heart defect. Don't worry, you'll have another." This took place over fifty years ago. I've proved her wrong.

This is my story. It is my journey as an adult living with a congenital heart defect. It is a story of pain, perseverance, and triumph and of denial, acceptance, and victory over congenital heart disease (CHD). And I am not alone. The estimated number of adults living with CHD—one million—equals or exceeds the number of children living with CHD.[1]

A Journey of the Heart

Learning to Thrive, Not Just Survive,
With Congenital Heart Disease

Deborah L. Flaherty-Kizer

Published by BookLocker.com, Inc., St. Petersburg, Florida.

Printed on acid-free paper.

Booklocker.com, Inc.
2017

First Edition

Dedication

This book is dedicated to Keith, my wonderful husband and the love of my life. You have been by my side every step of this journey. I couldn't have come this far without your love, encouragement, support, and laughter. You inspire me each day to live life fully and enjoy the journey!

Acknowledgements

This book would not have been possible without the love and support of my husband Keith and my wonderful children, Colin and Abby. Their encouragement helped make this book a reality.

I would like to thank the staff at Massachusetts General Hospital. Much thanks and gratitude go to my awesome cardiac surgeon, Dr. Thomas MacGillivray, whose superb surgical skills might only be surpassed by his compassionate care and sharp wit. I am grateful for my incredible adult congenital heart specialist, Dr. Ami Bhatt. Her keen sense of me as an individual, not just as a heart patient, gave—and continues to give—me much trust and confidence in her. Thanks also to wellness nurse Lauren MacLaughlin, who kindly met with Keith and me to provide some stress reduction and mindful breathing lessons. I can also never be thankful enough to the caring nurses and staff in the OR, the CICU, and the step down unit.

Closer to home, I owe my early recovery success to the caring team at Sunnyview Rehabilitation Hospital, particularly my lead physical therapist Kathryn Greene. Her encouragement and support helped me face each workout with a positive attitude. Many thanks as well to the wonderful nurses, doctors, and staff—even during my darkest moments they put a smile on my face.

To the St. Peter's Cardiac Rehabilitation and Wellness team, you are amazing! I don't know if I ached more from the exercise or the laughter. You encouraged and motivated me to stretch my limits.

Thanks also to my "home base" team of doctors, particularly Dr. Christopher Dibble of Cardiology Associates of Schenectady. His tenacity and determination helped ensure I received the care I needed and deserved. His parting advice after every appointment, to "keep swimming," encouraged me to press on. My appreciation goes to Dr. Michele Gorla, my pulmonologist. Our paths first crossed at Sunnyview and I am so grateful to him for getting me on the road to recovery. To my primary care physician, Dr. Nasrene Yadegari-Lewis, and phlebotomists Melissa and Michin—you became like family during my often several times a week Coumadin checks. Thanks also to Dr. Sara Clark, my endocrinologist—I am amazed by and grateful for her ability to look at the big picture. In addition, many thanks go to Dr. Puspa Das, my therapist, who helped me see the forest through the trees and stay positive.

I also offer deep appreciation to two wonderful organizations. To the staff of the Adult Congenital Heart Association and my fellow Heart to Heart Ambassadors, thank you for being a much-needed resource for adults living with congenital heart disease. To the

WomenHeart staff and my sister WomenHeart Champions, thank you for all you do to advocate for women's heart health. I very much appreciated the outreaches to me by both these organizations during this difficult time.

I would not be here today without the support, love, and prayers of many people. To my students at St. Madeleine Sophie School, thank you for the wonderful book you put together for me before I left for surgery. Thank you to the students and staff as well for your prayers and visits. I can't express enough gratitude to my dear friend, Pamela Wells—you have been riding along with me this whole trip. Thank you to a special group of individuals—Carolyn Kelly, Cindy Mosbey, and Marcy Winoker. I truly believe God brings people into your life when you need them most, and I thank you for your special roles in my pre- and post-surgery days. A special word of thanks goes to Coach Jenny Hadfield and the members of Coach Jenny's Challenge Facebook Group. Your concern, support, and motivation encouraged me and gave me strength more than you will ever know. Thanks also to my massage therapist, Lorraine Calleri, whose positive energy helped me stay positive. To my dear friend and yoga instructor Andrea Fortuin—thank you for showing me the benefits of yoga and Reiki massage pre- and post-surgery. Many, many thanks to the caring staff at Camp Bow Wow, who took wonderful care of Kovu while I was in the hospital.

Knowing he was being cared for and loved brightened my days.

Finally, I am thankful to God for getting me though this difficult time and for giving me the inspiration and ability to tell my story. I am truly blessed.

Table of Contents

Preface

Living with congenital heart disease is tough. Feeling alone with congenital heart disease is even tougher. There are more than 30 types of congenital heart diseases, and people with the same diagnosis can be at vastly different levels of health. One size does not fit all.

Growing up, I felt a sense of isolation with my undiagnosed congenital heart disease. Why couldn't I be as active as other kids were? Why did I continue to gain weight? No one I knew had a congenital heart problem, much less the rare defect I actually possessed. When at the age of 19 I was diagnosed with Ebstein's Anomaly, my whole world changed. What was the prognosis? Would I lead a normal life? I had more questions than answers.

I've discovered that I am truly able to thrive, not just survive, with congenital heart disease. It has led me on quite a journey, leading me to become an active volunteer, advocate, and spokesperson for women's heart health and congenital heart disease issues. I feel truly blessed to be able to use my disease to help others.

I never envisioned writing a book when I started keeping a journal about living with heart disease. I started journaling well before my open-heart surgery as a way to help me process what I was going through pre-surgery and would potentially be going through post-surgery. When I combined the writings about my pre- and post-surgery experiences and challenges, I realized I had quite a story to share with other heart patients.

On my heart journey, fellow congenital heart patients have encouraged me, motivated me, and shown me what is possible to accomplish even with a serious illness. I'm hoping this book reads like a conversation—one congenital heart patient sharing her journey with another, helping the reader realize that he or she is not alone with the worries and concerns that come with living with congenital heart disease. In some small way, my hope is that this book will inspire those living with congenital heart disease—or any illness—to also thrive, not just survive.

Growing Up

I never really considered myself as having a "disease." I knew I had something "wrong" with my heart, but I thought it wasn't anything major. All I knew was that I was overweight and was a total failure at all things athletic. Of course, back in the late 50s and early 60s, many girls did not worry so much about being physically fit. It seemed more important to be a raving beauty (which I was not), thin (which I was not), and tanned (being Irish, I definitely was not). I did excel academically, however. I convinced myself that a girl did not need to be athletic, that I could go far on brains alone. Well, that was true to a point, but I eventually discovered just how much my physical health would limit me.

Year after year, I would go for my annual pediatric check-up, year after year the doctor commented on my "galloping" heart, year after year he would tell my mother I needed to lose weight. No one had diagnosed exactly what was wrong—we were told it was just a "murmur." Medical technology was not that advanced back in those days.

As a teenager, I tried every fad diet there was, but without an exercise program, I was doomed to fail. It was a vicious cycle. I tired easily, so I figured I couldn't exercise. I didn't exercise, so I was always out of shape and heavy. I never linked my tiredness with my "murmur."

I never was under the care of a congenital heart specialist when I was young since the true extent of my heart disease was unknown. I was not treated "special," nor did I receive extra attention from my parents. Typical of doctor-patient relationships of that time, my parents accepted what my pediatrician told them and did not seek another medical opinion. Not knowing there was a medical reason for my lack of athletic prowess led to some self-esteem issues, as I just couldn't participate well in many childhood activities and felt like a failure. I dreaded gym class—I was always the last one picked for a team. I blamed myself. But at least I didn't have parents who coddled me or refused to let me do anything. My childhood might have been very different if doctors had diagnosed my heart condition when I was young. At any rate, focusing on academics was my only respite and motivator.

From the time I was in elementary school, I dreamed of attending one of the service academies. My father, a graduate of the United States Naval Academy and an instructor pilot, perished in a plane crash when I was only six months old. I wanted to attend a service academy as a way of honoring him. Never mind that women were not yet admitted. When the women's rights movement of the 60s opened up opportunities for women, I remember asking my mother if the academies would admit women. She said they never would.

Fast forward to 1975, my freshman year at college. I could not contain my excitement when I heard that women would be considered for appointments to the academies. I knew this meant I would have to restart my college experience if I was accepted, but to me it was worth it.

I immediately went through the application process and just waited. And waited. I found out my status in a most unusual way. Early one evening, I received a phone call. It was a reporter from the *Boston Globe*. I was one of the first women to receive an appointment to the U.S. Naval Academy and he would be at my house in 30 minutes to interview me! I was speechless, the only sound being my pounding heart. My mother moved through that house faster than the Energizer Bunny® to get it into white-glove shape. The reporter soon arrived with a photographer in tow to capture my story. I felt like I was dancing on a cloud. The next morning, I saw my story and photo on the front page of *the Boston Globe's* Living Section.

I had sailed through the academic requirements; only the physical fitness test and physical exam remained. I knew the fitness test would be difficult, but it was harder than I thought. Candidates had to do a set number of pull-ups, push-ups, and crunches and run a mile. Almost twenty years of no exercise took its toll, and the first time I took the physical fitness test, I failed miserably. My results weren't even close to what they needed to be. I was crushed. Determined to give it another try, I embarked on a physical fitness program designed to help me pass the "second chance" test. As a college student, I didn't have excess funds for gym memberships or trainers. I just used what I had available—extra gym classes that I could physically handle and the track. I even went so far as to use the shower bar for chin-ups. At first, I could barely do one, but within two months I was a chin-up champ, easily accomplishing seven!

The morning of the physical fitness test came around. I was nervous, but knew I had prepared myself to the best of my ability. I may never be a world-class athlete, but I felt I could conquer this mountain. And I did! I passed the test, and for the first time in my life, I felt physically strong. The only thing left was the mandatory physical exam.

It finally looked like my dream was coming true. My academy advisor called and gave me the news that I had been accepted pending the physical exam. In fact, he even said I had been assigned my roommate. He invited me to meet with him at his home, and we spent an entire afternoon discussing what life at the Naval Academy would be like. I couldn't have been happier. I remember him saying how thrilled he was for my appointment, and that it was about time women were admitted to the academies.

My ship soon sank. A few weeks later, my advisor called me, and I could sense he was upset. He told me that in spite of my passing the fitness test, in spite of my doctor saying I was physically able to attend the Academy, I had not passed the military physical. My acceptance had been rescinded because of my "condition." No specific diagnosis was mentioned, only that I should be seen by a congenital heart doctor because I had more than a murmur. I then realized that not being accepted into the Naval Academy was the least of my problems. I had no idea what I had wrong with me or how serious it was. My advisor assured me that if I wanted to fight the Academy's decision, he would be behind me 150 percent. I recognized that if I did, by the time I eventually entered the Academy I would have graduated college, so I cut my losses and moved on. I was devastated. I had never been discriminated against because of my illness; in fact, I didn't even know what condition I had! I was scared and frightened, and tried not to go to the "what if" place.

My quest to enter the academies led to my quest to uncover the nature of my heart ailment. I vowed then to do everything in my power to remain as healthy and fit as possible.

Knowledge is Power

I now knew that I had more than a murmur, but had no idea if my condition was life threatening. I felt I only had a partial diagnosis at this point. In fact, at this time the field of congenital cardiology was still relatively new. It was unlikely that my congenital heart disease could have been diagnosed when I was born in 1957. Until the 1940s, congenital heart disease was understood primarily from the landmark autopsy information compiled by Maude Abbott in 1924. Then, in 1947, the publication of *Congenital Malformations of the Heart* by Helen Taussig illuminated the clinical side of congenital heart disease.[2] With respect to my soon-to-be-diagnosed condition, Ebstein's Anomaly, during the 1960s, most attempts to repair the tricuspid valve were unsuccessful, and prosthetic valve replacement became the preferred approach. It wasn't until 1962 that Dr. Christian Barnard described the first successful tricuspid valve replacement in a patient with Ebstein's Anomaly using a mechanical valve.[3]

I was attending college in Weston, Massachusetts, about 30 minutes from home. I decided that the best place for me to be followed was Massachusetts General Hospital (MGH). I saw a congenital heart specialist there, Dr. Richard Liberthson, who informed me I have a rare congenital heart disease called Ebstein's Anomaly. Simply, in Ebstein's Anomaly, the tricuspid valve—the valve between the chambers on the right side of the heart—does not form correctly and thus doesn't work properly. Blood leaks back through the valve, making the heart work less efficiently. Ebstein's Anomaly may also lead to enlargement of the heart or heart failure. I was shocked—how could I have such a serious heart problem and not feel worse? How had I ever made it through the grueling Naval Academy physical fitness test?

Fortunately, at this point I did not require immediate surgery. I just needed to be monitored annually for any changes. There was only one caveat—I would need surgery if I wanted to bear children, as the strain on my untreated heart would be too great. Dr. Liberthson suggested that I consider adoption if I ever wanted children, since the surgery was risky and did not guarantee a successful pregnancy. I decided then and there that if the time came, adoption would be my choice.

Life Moves Along

After college and graduate school, I moved to New Jersey to begin my marketing career with AT&T. I still made my annual trip to Boston to see Dr. Liberthson. It was always good to return home and visit my parents for a few days. No changes to the plan—Dr. Liberthson told me to keep doing what I was doing. At this point, I had successfully gotten to my "goal weight" and felt great.

I had even found an exercise I loved—horseback riding. I started taking group lessons at the county stable and eventually took lessons at a private stable. I really enjoyed the discipline of dressage, the guiding of a horse through a series of complex maneuvers by slight movements of the rider's hands, legs, and weight. I was elated to find a sport I could excel in, and I loved competing in local horse shows. I was worry-free about my heart condition. After all, I was asymptomatic, on no medications, and felt fine.

I met my future husband Keith during the aftermath of a train wreck in New Jersey. I still worked for AT&T and Keith worked for ADT. It turned out we commuted to Manhattan on the same New Jersey Transit line. My commute was NJ Transit to Hoboken, then PATH to the World Trade Center, followed by a one-block walk to work. One cold February day in 1984, I arrived in Hoboken and entered into a huge crowd of commuters filling the station. PATH from Hoboken to Manhattan was down due to a train wreck! More trains were pulling into the station with loads of soon-to-be-unhappy commuters. A loudspeaker announcement noted that there were specially provided buses to Manhattan outside the station. There was no room for a mad dash. The best the desperate commuters could do was ooze towards the door for the buses. Another announcement then informed us that PATH was up from Harrison, New Jersey and there was a train loading on track 3 for Harrison. Anyone even close to track 3 was Harrison bound whether they wanted to go or not. I wasn't that close, but the oozing crowd carried me onto the train anyhow. Standing room only. Thankfully, it was a short ride to Harrison.

The Harrison PATH station is located several blocks away from the Harrison NJ Transit station, so our swarm of train commuters had to hoof it down the street through the cold misty morning to the PATH station. Exiting the station to begin the trek, I came across a scene from what could have been a Cecil B. DeMille production—as our group from the train flowed into the street toward the PATH station, another group came out of the mist toward us. PATH from Harrison was down as well!

Back on the train to return to Hoboken, this fellow started talking with me—a captive audience, I guess.

When we finally arrived at the World Trade Center (the PATH was operational by then), he asked me out to lunch. I told him since it was almost 11:00 a.m. I should probably show up at work. He asked for my number. I noticed that he didn't write it down, so I didn't think anything would come of it. Was I surprised when he called me at work early the next morning to invite me to lunch! Such was our first date.

It's always a risky decision to tell a potential significant other about a major health issue. A few months into our relationship, I decided it was time to tell him about my heart disease and the related issues and constraints. Better to have an early failure, I figured, than invest too much in a relationship that might not go anywhere because of my condition. Turned out, it was not a deal breaker. Keith, too, had some medical baggage. A shooting accident when he was a teenager injured his spinal cord so he walked with a cane.

Three years after our wedding, we were blessed with the adoption of our son, Colin. We brought him home when he was just five weeks old. The day we found out we had a son was quite an interesting one. Keith had planned to help me at a dressage competition, but ended up having to work because of a computer system problem. "Of all days," I complained to him. I really hated going to shows alone, but I decided to go anyway. I couldn't believe when my horse Jubi and I took first place! Jubi was an old former school pony who had only one eye. Competitors riding thoroughbreds would look at us with one eyebrow raised, but they were subsequently dumbfounded when Jubi would usually win or place. On this day, however, a rider on an elegant thoroughbred and her mom came over to us. "Is that Jubi?" the mom asked. When I said it was, a big smile broke out on her face. "My daughter learned to ride on Jubi," she said, "and now she is trying out for the U.S. Equestrian Team." She gave Jubi a welcome treat. My day kept getting better and better!

I returned home and couldn't wait to share my day with Keith. Much was my surprise when the doorbell rang and it was Keith—had he lost his keys? I noticed he was holding a floral arrangement with a baby boy balloon attached. "Who are these for?" I asked, thinking that maybe someone at his work had given birth.

"The adoption agency called," he said. "These are for you." That was one day I will never forget!

About five months later, Colin was sick, and Keith agreed to stay home with him in the morning. I would relieve him at lunchtime. When I returned home and walked into the house, I was shocked by what I saw. Our dining room table was set with fine china, champagne, and a bouquet of flowers. All I could think was what did Keith do now? He very slowly explained that he had received a call from the adoption agency asking if we would consider adopting a soon-to-bearriving birth sibling. After Keith picked me up off the floor, we discussed it and agreed to adopt again! Baby Abigail joined our family several months later.

Fortunately, I was able to take advantage of an early retirement offer from AT&T, enabling me to stay home with our children. Since the package also included money for tuition, I went back to a nearby college to earn a master's degree in elementary education. That way, when Colin and Abby eventually went to school, I had the option of teaching in a local school with the same schedule.

Even with our health limitations, Keith and I always tried to model a healthy lifestyle for our children. At this point, we had relocated to upstate New York, so it was easy to take advantage of outdoor activities. I took them cross-country skiing in winter and swimming to a nearby lake in summer. We would often go to Five Rivers Environmental Educational Center and hike their trails.

One of my favorite activities to do with my daughter was ballet. I had taken ballet as a child and decided that rather than sit in the waiting room during her many classes at Albany Berkshire Ballet, I would join her in class. I ended up becoming sort of an assistant to Miss Madeleine, the ballet mistress, especially during recital time. I even went on tour with the Nutcracker, playing a sword-wielding mouse to Abby's soldier. Abby and I also participated in many master's classes with several New York City Ballet principal dancers while they were in nearby Saratoga Springs for their annual summer residency at the Saratoga Performing Arts Center. Such wonderful memories!

With raising children and everyday life, I got out of the practice of making my annual pilgrimage to MGH, now a three-hour drive. After all, I felt fine and thought I couldn't afford the time off from work—I had started teaching at our parish school, St. Madeleine Sophie—or away from family. Eventually, this lack of specialized congenital care caught up with me. I thought I could get by just seeing my local cardiologist at the time, Dr. Douglas Long, for my annual checkup. However, Dr. Long said that I really should be followed again by a congenital heart specialist. He recommended MGH—right back where I started! As the number of adults with CHD has grown—and these adults are living longer thanks to medical technology—so has the need to have them followed by congenital cardiologists trained to treat adults, not children. As we age, we often present with a bucketful of other health issues. I can vouch for that! I now see enough specialized doctors to field a football team.

So back to Boston I went. My new adult congenital cardiologist, Dr. Ami Bhatt, was actually taking over the practice from Dr. Liberthson, whom I had seen as a young adult. Her knowledge, dedication, and commitment immediately impressed me. Everything seemed fine, but she did raise the issue of surgery "down the road." I hoped the road was long.

Taking Control

I finally admitted to myself that I had not been taking control of my life or myself. The 25 pounds I had lost in my twenties had crept back and then some—an additional 25 pounds! I reached the realization that while I am a control freak for others, I do not impose the same rigidity on myself. I had my wake-up call after going through months of up-and-down weight loss, always stuck on the high end. Due to a nasty fall off our horse Poco, I could no longer ride, so my exercise efforts had come to a standstill. I blamed sleep apnea, thyroid issues, caretaking responsibilities, etc., but finally realized the responsibility was mine and mine alone. I tried not to berate myself with "stinkin' thinkin'," but recognized if the fault lies with me, so does the fix. I found it all too easy to blame the stressors in my life—terminally ill mother, two young adults still living at home, a stressful teaching job—you name it, I could call it an excuse.

It took a trio of events to get me serious about making positive lifestyle changes. First was a trip to the Ellis Hospital Emergency Room. I woke up one Saturday with extremely sharp shoulder and chest pain. Ignoring my advice to others to call 911 if you experience any heart attack symptoms, I had Keith drive me to the hospital. I was petrified—I truly didn't think I was having a heart attack, but if I was, I was concerned that the hospital would not know what to do given my congenital issue. Once in a room, I was swarmed by many medical professionals who inserted an IV, drew blood, and took my vitals. Fortunately, the ER doctor on-call decided to bring in a cardiologist to look over the test results. Although he didn't think I was having a cardiac incident, he wanted me to stay overnight for observation. That was enough to scare some sense into me—the last thing I wanted was to need some sort of procedure.

The second kick in my pants I needed to get me moving towards a healthier lifestyle was the death of my mother on June 8, 2012. She had begun to fail around the spring of 2011. My parents moved in with us soon after that. My mom was suffering from dementia, and as we would soon find out, lung cancer. She had been a heavy smoker all her life, and she was now paying the price. Unfortunately, along with her dementia came extreme paranoia. Every week seemed to bring a trip to the ER.

Eventually she was admitted into a psychiatric facility, which then released her to a nursing home that could not meet her needs. To yet another hospital she went, where she stayed until her death. Increasingly, my mother became mean, defiant, and unwilling to see any family. I found this extremely difficult to bear, as I had done so much for her, and her telling me to "get out of here you fat ugly thing" shook me to the core.

I know my mom had many regrets in her life and lived it for others, not herself. When she died, I vowed I would get myself healthy and put my health and my needs first. I've learned this is not being selfish; rather, how could I take care of my family and give my best in any endeavor if I was not well?

The third event was a trip to a cardiac surgeon in June of 2012. At my appointment with Dr. Bhatt in early 2012, she noted that there was some deterioration of my heart function. She wanted me to meet with her recommended surgeon, Dr. Thomas MacGillivray, to discuss the possibility of surgery. I remember it well. We met with Dr. MacGillivray exactly two weeks after my mother died. Thank goodness, Keith accompanied me, as I was still numb from my mother's passing. In our meeting with Dr. MacGillivray, he presented us with two surgical options—fixing the tricuspid valve or replacing it with a tissue valve. Dr. MacGillivray gently but strongly urged me to drop some 50 pounds and get into better shape—the healthier I was going into surgery the better the outcome and recovery would be. After my earlier stint in Ellis, I wanted to spend the least amount of time in the hospital as possible. While no surgery was scheduled, I sensed the exit for the road to surgery was approaching.

Once life seemed to go back to normal (or as normal as possible) after my mom's death, I realized that I had an entire summer pretty much to myself. No running to doctors, hospitals, or appointments with my mom and dad. No cooking for what seemed like 24 hours a day, no multiple loads of laundry—I felt free! I vowed to target that summer as the one when I would get serious about my weight and health. The pink elephant had been in the living room for far too long. I acknowledged that it had taken time for me to get to this point, and it would take time and commitment to reverse it. I needed to hold myself accountable for my actions. My first step was to rejoin Weight Watchers with my good friend Pam. We both had had the "year from hell" and decided to make the commitment and effort to get back in shape. It was—and still is—harder than I thought!

I also recommitted to an exercise program, now having the luxury of being home over the summer. During the school year, after being on my feet teaching all day, the last place I felt like heading to at the end of the day was the gym. During that summer, I tried to swim 40 laps at least four times per week and walk every day. I even took boxing lessons! If I was to stick to any type of exercise routine, it had to be fun and challenging.

While at the Y, I saw a notice for the indoor triathlon, which consists of a 15-minute swim, followed by a 15-minute stationary bike ride, and ending with a 15-minute walk or run on the treadmill. "Boy, I wish I could do that," I thought to myself. But there was no way—I was too fat, too untrained, and too non-athletic. I let that opportunity slip away. The next year however, I said what the heck—I signed up not having a clue what to expect. I also signed up my son so he could complete his final badge requirement to make Eagle Scout. Now I had a training partner! We both had an amazing time working out together.

Due to his work schedule, Colin needed an earlier start time for the triathlon. Normally the older entrants get the early times, probably because the younger set likes to sleep in. The Y allowed Colin and me to switch times. In the first event, the swim, Colin ended up being with competitors in the 50+-age bracket. He looked like Michael Phelps compared with them! I, however, was not so lucky. My group consisted of seven strapping young men in Speedos and me. The men were tearing up the pool, but I think my lap counter could have gone out for breakfast I was so slow. But I did it! Colin and I both made it through the bike and treadmill portions with no problem. We were triathletes!

Participating in this annual event has become a tradition for me now. It doesn't even bother me that I usually come in last place—I am really only competing against myself. Each year, Keith gladly serves as my cheerleader and wingman, encouraging me every step of the way. He also makes sure I have enough water, and he sets up the bike for me before my heat starts. Most importantly, when I'm done, he takes my worn-out body to our favorite diner for breakfast. The YMCA staff as well supports and cheers everyone on. It has become my favorite event.

It's Time

The boom was lowered at my November of 2014 annual appointment with Dr. Bhatt. She announced, "It's time." I assumed she didn't mean lunch, but surgery. Unfortunately, I was right. In my heart, I too knew that it was time. Daily activities such as climbing stairs were starting to become a struggle. I have to say though that I was probably failing a little bit each year, and it was just at the point of becoming noticeable to me. I was exhausted every afternoon after school. My legs and feet were becoming more swollen more often.

Determining the appropriate need and time for congenital heart surgery seems to be part art, part science. It only took a simple walk around Dr. Bhatt's office with a pulse oximeter (it measures your oxygen levels) for her to say it was time. When I asked her when, she replied, "Whenever you want within the next two years!" I was surprised. Unlike other heart surgeries that can occur in an emergency, congenital heart surgery is often something you can plan for ahead of time, giving you the opportunity to get as prepared as possible. I asked her if May of 2015 would be OK, and she agreed. My plan was to be home by Memorial Day and enjoy the summer taking walks and sitting out on the deck. Additionally, my son and his fiancée,

Krissy, were planning their wedding for May of 2016, so I wanted to make sure I was dance floor ready!

My husband and I met again with my surgeon, Dr. MacGillivray, in February of 2015, during Boston's snowiest season on record. Talk about a winter wonderland! Ice and immensely high snow banks made the quick walk from our hotel to the hospital impossible. We relied on door-to-door taxi service.

I came prepared with my list of questions and concerns. I had actually emailed them to his physician's assistant the week before so they could be addressed. She helped direct me to the proper organizations for questions the surgeon or she could not answer. I found it very helpful to have Keith at the meeting with me. He was able to take notes and ask other questions. Dr. MacGillivray posed several seemingly simple questions to me, such as how I was tolerating exercise and how many hours I slept each night, which helped him assess the state of my heart. When he questioned me as to how I felt, I noted that I was tired at day's end from chasing after a rambunctious second grade class all day. "Well," he said, "that would tire even Tom Brady out." Ah, how Bostonians love their sports!

At this point, Dr. MacGillivray had a surgical game plan. He would replace the tricuspid valve with a porcine valve, close up an atrial septal defect (hole), and perform a bidirectional Glenn shunt procedure. In this procedure, the superior vena cava is divided from the right atrium and moved from the right atrium to the pulmonary artery. This allows deoxygenated "blue" blood from the head to drain passively to lungs. I was relieved that he was opting for a tissue rather than a mechanical valve replacement, as I would not have to take a blood thinner for life. When I asked if there were any alternatives to surgery, he seriously noted, "Well, you could be looking at a heart transplant down the road otherwise." That was not a road I wanted to take.

While there are some basic questions you need to ask (see Appendix), how much detail you want to know about the actual surgical procedure is up to you and what you think you can emotionally handle. Some people want to know every detail, watch videos of prior surgeries, etc., while others just want the high-level overview. I just wanted the main facts; Keith wanted the details. So, after we both talked with Dr. MacGillivray, Keith discussed all the details with him while I spoke with his assistant in another room about more general topics, such as ways to prepare for surgery, expected time in the hospital, and recovery milestones.

You should also be given the opportunity to speak with an anesthesiologist. Ask to meet with one if it is not suggested. This is the time to discuss any particular concerns you may have about what and how much anesthesia will be used, its effects, and any other issues. If you want the anesthesiologist to read positive affirmations before your surgery, be sure to ask if this is possible. I mentioned this when I met with an anesthesiologist, and he said there would be no problem. I would just need to have someone give my attending anesthesiologist the affirmations when they took me to the operating room. I used the affirmations from Peggy Huddleston's book <u>Prepare for Surgery, Heal Faster</u> and made sure Keith had them to hand over at the appropriate time.

Ongoing, proper dental care is crucial for any heart patient. While research has found a link between heart disease and gum disease, it's not clear whether one actually causes the other, according to the American Heart Association. One hypothesis is that bacteria from the oral cavity spread throughout the body, worsening other inflammatory conditions, like heart disease, rheumatoid arthritis, and type 2 diabetes.[4]

Depending on your condition, you may need to take antibiotics before any routine dental prophylaxis (cleaning) to reduce the risk for infective endocarditis, an infection of the heart's lining or valves. The guidelines did change a few years ago, so it's best to check with your cardiologist. Your insurance may also cover three dental prophylaxes a year versus the usual two, again depending on your specific heart disease.

It is best to have any major dental work, such as tooth extractions, done well before any heart surgery. In a small, retrospective study, Mayo Clinic researchers found that 8% of heart patients who had teeth pulled close to surgery suffered major adverse health outcomes, such as a heart attack, stroke, kidney failure, or death.[5] I started experiencing decay in my wisdom teeth several years before I thought I would probably be having heart surgery. Knowing this, my dentist recommended having them pulled well before the surgery to avoid further decay, any inflammation, or complications after heart surgery. I certainly did not want to put off my surgery because of a dental issue! I agreed with this proactive approach and had all four extracted (ugh).

It's a good idea to have a dental prophylaxis and tooth x-rays done before heart surgery as well. MGH required a signoff from my dentist to clear me for surgery from a dental standpoint. Also, Dr. MacGillivray wanted me to wait six months after surgery before having my teeth cleaned again, so I made sure that I had a cleaning a month or so before surgery.

We set May 21, 2015 as the surgery date. It fit in with my plan perfectly, as I wanted to be home by Memorial Day weekend. Dr. MacGillivray suggested I do as much exercise as I could tolerate to prepare myself. I got the sense that the surgery was complicated, but that it was routine for him. After all, I thought, Dr. Bhatt wouldn't send me to someone she didn't trust. Now came the hard part—preparing myself physically, emotionally, and spiritually for surgery.

It can be helpful to seek out a second or even third opinion if that makes you feel comfortable. Many well-known congenital heart centers will review your case electronically—you don't even need to travel to their facility. Insurance may or may not cover the review, but it might be worth peace of mind. I must admit that I did not seek a second opinion. I knew that my condition was rare and that there were probably only a handful of surgeons with enough experience and expertise to perform the surgery. Looking back, I know I made the right decision, and that for me having too many options would have caused more stress. My care at MGH was excellent, and the post-surgery visit during the tough initial recovery period was relatively easy to manage. I know I would have had a difficult time flying across country or driving more than five hours for this visit given my post-surgery condition.

Dr. Bhatt asked if I was willing to talk with a patient who went through a somewhat similar surgery at MGH, and I jumped at the chance. Thankfully, the patient was willing to talk with me and met Keith and me for lunch at the hospital during one of my pre-surgery visits. Hearing her story and seeing her so healthy further validated my choice. She, too, had not sought another opinion, noting that "People come all over the world for care here—there's no better place."

It's Starting to Get Real

Physically, I tried to exercise as much as I could tolerate so I would be in the best shape possible before surgery. I was starting to tire more easily—my 40 lap swims became only 20 laps, and I walked Kovu a half mile instead of a full one. My favorite event, the YMCA's indoor triathlon, was scheduled for two months before surgery. I was on the fence about participating until two "coaches" persuaded me to go for it. Cindy, the aquatics coordinator at the Y, reminded me I could go at my own pace and that the main goal was to have fun. A member of Coach Jenny's Challenge, the online Facebook exercise group I had joined, urged me to participate and use my time as a baseline for future post-surgery triathlons. I signed up. Given my decrease in exercise tolerance, my goal was just to finish. I not only posted times equivalent to the prior years' times, but for the first time in any Y event, I wasn't the last place finisher!

Nutritionally, I removed processed foods from my diet. I became a serious label reader and discovered that many items, although low calorie and high fiber, contain far too much sodium. In looking at an item's ingredients, I figured that if I couldn't pronounce it, it probably wasn't good for me. I began preparing foods simply, avoiding sauces and butter, and started leaving fruit out in a bowl for quick snacks. I also joined a community supported agriculture program. Each week I receive a bag of farm-fresh vegetables and fruit. I've tried veggies I had never heard of, such as kohlrabi, celery root, fiddleheads, and purslane. Easy recipes are also provided. Every week it's like Christmas morning. I can't wait to open the bag!

I had a tough time dealing with the pre-surgery emotional rollercoaster ride. I worried about everything—will I even make it to surgery, will I make it through the operation, how will I feel? Interestingly, I never worried about dying—I was more concerned that I would have a stroke and end up paralyzed.

I drove myself crazy with the "what ifs." I second-guessed my choice of hospital and surgeon. Should I have asked for another opinion, should I have gone somewhere else? Rationally, I knew I had made the right choice—granted, I had been followed at MGH for years as a teen and adult. But I still had my doubts. It was like premarital jitters. Dr. Bhatt must have a sixth sense—she contacted me right when I was experiencing all these worries and put my mind to rest. She emphasized that if she thought there was a better surgeon or hospital for me, she would have recommended that. (I actually found a patient for whom she did recommend a different hospital, which for some reason made me feel better.) She reassured me that Dr. MacGillivray was imminently knowledgeable about not only my condition but with me—he had been following my case for several years. Dr. MacGillivray has been a surgeon for over 20 years, and was featured in *Boston Magazine*[6] in 2006. In the article, his colleague Dr. Gus Vlahakes noted, "Dr. MacGillivray can walk into a complex situation and know exactly what to do, even when there is no one around to consult with. He has an encyclopedic knowledge of the medical literature, and he pours an extensive amount of time into patient care. He doesn't shy away from the tough cases." I felt I was in competent hands.

I was also seeing a therapist, Dr. Puspa Das, for my pre-surgery anxiety. I finally took to heart that there are things I can control and things I can't. I needed to learn to distinguish between the two and work on what I could control. To manage stress, I started taking yoga and practicing meditation. I had a monthly massage to help reduce stress and anxiety. A practicing Catholic, I believe in the power of prayer and faith. I also feel that sometimes I have to "let go and let God." Giving my surgery and healing over to God was a great release of the heavy burden I felt.

I also discovered that MGH had launched the Adult Congenital Heart Disease Health and Wellness Program, which provides patients with stress management techniques including in-appointment meditation and yoga, nutrition counseling, food diaries, and setting exercise and weight loss goals. Fortunately, I was able to meet one of the Wellness Center nurses, Lauren McLaughlin, during a pre-surgery visit. She gave me some good, practical techniques for dealing with stress and anxiety, including meditation and counted deep breathing techniques. Simple breathing exercises can truly help lower stress and anxiety. Keith actually still uses them during stressful driving situations!

While each person's experience with CHD is unique, you may find it helpful to talk to someone who has been or is currently in a similar medical situation. The Adult Congenital Heart Association's Heart to Heart Ambassador Program offers members of ACHA and their families the opportunity to connect one-on-one with an ACHA ambassador in a positive, supportive way. Ambassadors, who are either individuals with CHD or a relative of someone with CHD, provide support, guidance, and resources.

Hopping through the Health Insurance Hoop

The ACHA and other leading heart organizations recommend that adults with congenital heart disease be monitored at specialized adult congenital heart disease centers. Oftentimes, these are not located in the same health insurance network as the patient. If you are going to a hospital or center your insurance views as "out of network," start the insurance authorization process early. My insurer denied the initial request to have my surgery at MGH—I was told there were plenty of pediatric congenital cardiac surgeons in my area. Really? I was 57 years old! Thank goodness for my local cardiologist, Dr. Christopher Dibble, who sent my insurer a letter stating that the surgery I required was not performed at any local hospital. Within days, my insurer approved the surgery and follow-up visits.

It really annoys me that I have to go through this approval process every year when I visit MGH for my annual checkup. Yes, I know insurers are worried about insurance fraud. However, it's not as if my condition is miraculously going to disappear. What I would like to see is a blanket five or 10-year approval for such congenital issues, allowing patients to visit "out-of-network" providers at a frequency recommended by their CHD cardiologist. Living with congenital heart disease is stressful enough without having to deal with insurance issues.

Boston, Here We Come

How quickly the time flew! On May 19, Keith and I headed up to Boston for the big event. Although it seems silly, one of the hardest things I had to do was to drop off our dog Kovu at Camp Bow Wow. I gave him a big hug and promised him I would be back soon. How long would it be, I wondered, before we could take walks again through the beautiful Pine Bush Preserve?

Colin and Krissy were planning to come up the day before surgery. My daughter Abby, who lives in Florida, promised to pray for me and send healing thoughts. I tried not to let my mind wander to dark places—I knew the importance of staying positive and realized that doing so was my only option at this point.

Before leaving for Boston, I set up contact people who could relay information about my condition to friends and family. I did not want to burden Keith with having to make calls or send emails. Social media proved to be very helpful in this regard—Keith just gave status reports to Abby and select friends in the closed Facebook groups I belonged to and they in turn posted the updates.

I also did the tasks one typically does before going away, such as have the mail held and cancel the newspaper. Since I pay most of our bills electronically, I made sure payments due for the rest of May and June were scheduled. I also made up a list of websites and passwords for Keith in case he needed access to any accounts.

I often am asked how much information I gave my children about my operation. From the time they could understand my heart issue, both Colin and Abby knew I had CHD. We often felt like characters in a sitcom—Keith with his cane, me with my heart, and the two adopted siblings. Although Colin and Abby were in their twenties by the time I had surgery, I gave them just a top-level overview of what would happen. I let them decide whether or not they wanted to come to Boston for the surgery and let them know that I would be OK with their decision. I admit I was concerned when my son said he would be there because I had terrible memories of seeing my own mother in the cardiac intensive care unit (CICU) soon after her heart surgery and found the experience quite disconcerting. In fact, the nurse had to get me a chair since I thought I was going to faint. However, with Colin's Eagle Scout training, I knew he could handle it. I was glad that he and Krissy would be there not only to support me, but to comfort Keith as well. I remember feeling so alone and helpless during my mother's surgery—I was the only one there for her in the waiting room.

I did not want to burden my children or have them worry excessively. I'd heard about pre-surgery patients writing "In case of death" letters to each of their loved ones, but I could not bring myself to do this. For some reason, it seemed like tempting fate and tore me away from keeping an upbeat and positive attitude. I did, however, indulge myself and spent a weekend in Florida with Abby about a month before surgery. Since she couldn't come up for the surgery, I wanted to be sure we had some dedicated mother/daughter time.

If you are struggling with what and how much to tell your children, my advice is to keep the discussion age appropriate. What you tell a six-year-old is different from what you would tell a 17-year-old. The main thing is to tell your children that they will be safe, cared for, and loved during your surgery and recovery. For younger children, you may want to explain that it might be some time before you can play with them or lift them. Also, consider what each child can emotionally handle. Again, I felt more comfortable having my son there for my surgery than my daughter. While I didn't think the sight of me in the CICU would bother Colin, I thought it would disturb Abby.

I packed the loosest-fitting clothes I had to take to the hospital. Because of post-cardiac surgery fluid retention, you can expect to gain weight. I brought some things from home to put on my hospital wall—a favorite card from Abby and my bib from the indoor triathlon I had done in March. I also brought the scrapbook of cards my second graders had made for me.

It's often the smallest thing that means so much. I had become Facebook friends with Marcy, a member of Coach Jenny's Challenge Group. It turns out we had a lot in common—she lived in the Boston area and worked at the small Catholic high school I attended. We had been trying to get together during some of my earlier trips to the hospital, but things never worked out. It just so happened that the Thai restaurant I was eager to try was right across the street from where we were staying. Marcy met us there for dinner. What a wonderful time we had! It was like God sent an angel to us—having an upbeat and warm dining experience the night before I was admitted took our minds off what was to come. We talked and talked as if we had known each other for years. We discussed training plans, work, family—everything upbeat and positive. Sharing a meal took some of the burden off Keith. It would not have been good for either of us to be by ourselves mulling over the unknown challenges coming my way.

My MGH Experience

I must have been extremely stressed because I remember very little about the time leading up to surgery. The day before surgery I had a cardiac catheterization. I was a nervous wreck—my veins are extremely hard to access, so blood draws and IV placements are never quick and easy. (I always inform the medical staff of this so they can use a smaller needle.) I remember going into the catheterization lab and being greeted by some kind and caring technicians, doctors, and nurses. And that is about all.

One thing I do remember was a doctor telling me my arteries were clear as a bell. I had been surprised to find out that having a congenital heart problem does not give you a "get out of jail free" card for acquired heart disease. It seemed my lifestyle changes had paid off.

I was one of Dr. MacGillivray's "Thursday specials," which meant I was the only operation on his schedule. Thursdays were reserved for his most complicated and time-consuming cases. While this knowledge troubled me somewhat, I trusted that I was in extremely capable hands.

Surgery day dawned much too bright and early for me. I had spent the night at the hospital and was hoping for an early start time so I wouldn't have time to get anxious. It wasn't until about 9:30 a.m. when I was finally wheeled down to the operating suite. I remember waving to Keith, Colin, and Krissy as they took me away. Keith said I looked like a little ship sailing off, my eyes focused ahead. Things were foggy at this point as I had already been give some medication—I remember seeing people on my right near the operating room, but that's about it. Keith had given the orderly the positive affirmations I wanted read over me, such as "The surgery went well, you are on your way to healing," but I don't recall if they were read. I had also requested that classical music (nothing dark!) be playing before and during surgery, but I don't remember hearing anything. I had been told that I would be in the operating room for at least six hours. The procedure itself, however, would take about two hours. Much of the time is spent before and after the actual surgery—opening and closing the sternum, connecting and disconnecting the heart-lung machine, and monitoring vitals. Dr. MacGillivray's surgical plan remained as we had discussed—replace my tricuspid valve, close a hole in my heart, and perform a bidirectional Glenn shunt procedure.

When I first came to, everything seemed foggy. I struggled to communicate with others after the nurse removed the breathing tube. Every movement and even speaking seemed to take an extraordinary amount of effort. I realized I couldn't touch my fingers together or lift my arms. Because of all the fluid pumped into me during surgery, I had gained over 20 pounds. I remember being back in the operating room, seeing a doctor to my left, and hearing him say "We need platelets." Fortunately, Dr. MacGillivray was still there—it was now close to midnight—and he was able to fix the problem, which I later found out was a leaking blood vessel.

I cannot recall many events or their sequence during this time. When I later asked Dr. Bhatt's intern about this memory gap, she smiled and said it was by design. Evidently, I had been given some strong medications. I vaguely remember at some point that Keith was talking to one of the nurses and I was trying to get his attention. I was thirsty and wanted ice chips—my only possible, when allowed, "food." I still could not move a muscle so I could not get his attention. So out popped my first post-surgery words: "Shut up!" That got his attention. Keith told me later that everyone had a good laugh. I don't remember moving to the step down unit. I do recall Colin and Krissy visiting at one point with an adorable stuffed lion for me, and I remember the lovely flowers sent by Keith's coworkers. I also remember receiving, but not when, a beautiful plant from the ACHA (which is now in my family room and reminds me of what I have been through) and a delightful box of assorted teas (which I greatly enjoyed during recovery) from WomenHeart.

I also remember that the things I had worried about most before surgery proved to be inconsequential. One of my biggest concerns had been how I would deal with the removal of all the tubes and temporary pacemaker wires. I had been stressing over this for months before surgery; I was sure it would be painful. Turned out to be a non-issue. At one point, Dr. MacGillivray himself came in to remove the wires. We chatted for a bit, and I asked him to let me know when he was going to remove the wires. He said he would count down from five and asked me, "Are you ready?" I said I thought so, and with a smile on his face he remarked, "I removed those five minutes ago." Love that wit!

Even a week after surgery, I was very unsteady on my feet. At one point, I needed a chest x-ray to assess the fluid level in my lungs. The technician asked me to stand and hold on to the handles on the sides of the machine. After about five seconds, I could feel myself slipping. "Help!" I yelled, and proceeded to continue my downward slide only to collapse onto the men who had rushed in to assist me. The impact was so great we landed on the floor. Taking the x-ray while I was in my chair worked much better! When I returned to my room, a nurse asked me how it went. "Well," I replied, "nothing like an afternoon romp on the floor." Everyone broke into laughter, except Keith who looked horrified. This non-ambulatory state continued—I almost took down the health aide when she tried to help me with my first shower. Fortunately, at this point, I was not experiencing any pain in my chest or at the incision—I was still on some strong painkillers.

Laughter was my saving grace and I was blessed to have a wonderful roommate in Edie. Because I could not lay flat in bed, I spent most of the time in my hospital chair, which was fine by me. However, during mealtime, the tray somewhat blocked the access to the bathroom. Edie got up to use the bathroom. Let's just say she didn't make it through the obstacle course in time. I rang for the nurse and merely said "Cleanup in aisle 8." Edie and I laughed so hard I think she went again. It was wonderful to have someone around my age to laugh and share stories with—it helped the time go by. I had the pleasure of seeing Edie and her delightful husband Bill 10 months post-surgery in Florida.

The kindness, support, encouragement, and professionalism of those who attended to my care amazed me. They not only provided physical support, but emotional support as well. At one point before surgery, I felt overwhelmed by it all—one nurse just calmly sat with me and held my hand. I will never forget the nurses clapping and calling out words of encouragement as I made my first post-surgery walk in the corridor with my physical therapist. I felt like I had just completed a marathon! They took the time to know me as a person, not just a patient. In my room, my husband had taped up my racing bib from the indoor triathlon I had completed two months before. I wanted it there to motivate me and remind me of what I had overcome. One of the nurses asked me about it, and come to find out she was a triathlete. Talking about something I love brought back many happy memories and was a great distraction from the hospital routine. It also motivated me to keep up my daily walks. I was so thrilled when I made it around the floor "loop."

I was blessed to have several non-family visitors during my stay. Two friends from high school, Maureen and Ellie, stopped by. We hadn't seen each other for years but we picked up right where we had left off. It felt like we were back in high school, dishing up news of our former classmates. My Challenger friend Marcy and her boyfriend Ben visited as well. It was great just to talk with others and receive their encouragement.

Dr. McGillivray and Dr. Bhatt thought I would be in the hospital for five to seven days. One week turned into two and I was still there. My oxygen saturation level was still low, my heartbeat was somewhat erratic, and I was still retaining excess fluid. We discussed options—continued hospitalization, rehabilitation in Massachusetts, or rehabilitation back home in New York. We decided that I should be admitted into a rehabilitation facility. I wanted to be admitted to one close to home if possible. Fortunately, the hospital staff secured the necessary insurance approvals for me for transport and admittance to a facility in Schenectady, New York, about 30 minutes from home. Although I could sit up, eat, drink and had no IVs, I still had issues with stamina and mobility. Traveling home by car was out of the question. Rest stop restrooms presented a particular challenge; there was no way, being 22 pounds over my pre-surgery weight and having walked a maximum of 75 feet with a physical therapist, that I had even a prayer of walking to a restroom. With Keith's mobility issues, he would certainly have had a tough time picking me up off the floor. Having Keith drive me was just not an option.

Once the transfer date was set, Keith returned home to get the house in order and retrieve Kovu. Although the hotel he stayed in while I was in the hospital provides a discounted hospital rate, it had turned into a much longer and more expensive trip than we had planned. He was ready to return home.

Off to Sunny View

I was ready to leave! On June 5, I was loaded onto a stretcher and made my final wave to the floor nurses and staff. I didn't make the connection until a year later that my discharge date was my daughter's birthday! What happened next was the most god-awful ride of my life. Nothing like four hours in an ambulance with a bar pushing against your spine. I had eaten a light breakfast and did not want to eat or drink anything. The last thing I wanted to do was negotiate a bathroom break. I should have taken pain medication before the trip as well—everything ached after the first hour.

Hallelujah! We finally arrived at Sunnyview. By this time, I felt like a three-year-old on a long car trip. I was tired, cranky, and hungry. I had not had anything to eat or drink since breakfast. It seemed to take forever to get through the admission procedure. It all seemed surreal—I wished Keith had been there to help me wade through the paperwork and answer the seemingly endless number of questions. It was after 3:00 p.m. when I finally got to my room. Thank goodness, the ambulance drivers must have told a nurse that I hadn't had lunch. An angel came in with a deli plate for me. I could have kissed her. Soon after, Keith arrived with my dear friend Pam. Was I happy to see them! Pam hadn't seen me since before surgery and we greeted each other with tears and hugs. Our friendship began when our boys were in Boy Scouts. We have been there for each other many times—my dad and mom's illnesses, her husband and dad's passings, and my mom's passing. We've shared our weight loss ups and downs.

What followed next were three long and sometimes agonizing weeks at Sunnyview. At times, it was almost unbearable. The minutes turned into hours, the hours into days, and the days into weeks. I hated waking up each morning and facing the daily blood draw. I am a very difficult stick, and it usually took four different phlebotomists, each taking two or three tries, before my blood was successfully drawn. I still had a large amount of excess fluid, which added to the difficulty. They ended up sending in the ER nurse from the attached hospital, Ellis, who was experienced in difficult blood draws. Since she too had difficulty, a midline was inserted into my arm, which worked for about a week. Then back to the old poke and stick.

I did enjoy having a daily routine. Each morning I received a schedule for dressing, bathing, physical therapy, occupational therapy, and daily walk. On the first day, my lead therapist, Kathryn, had me do a benchmark walk—I barely made it down the hall. I knew I had a long way to go, but at least I was up and moving more—a noticeable change from my hospital days.

During physical therapy, we would work on building my strength and stamina. I really enjoyed using the Nu-Step recumbent trainer. I could actually see progress—I started with five-minute sessions but by the end of my time at Sunnyview I was up to 20 minutes! We also worked on negotiating a single step with a walker.

I was still on sternal precautions. Sternal precautions help prevent the separation of your breastbone as it heals. Separation of your sternum may slow the healing process of the bone. Sternal precautions also help to prevent excessive pulling on the surgical incision and keep the skin closed to prevent infection in your incision[7]. Fortunately, I was not experiencing any pain at the incision, but I still had to follow the precautions for a few months. My precautions included no lifting more than five pounds, no pushing or pulling with my arms, no reaching behind my back or reaching both arms out to the side, and no reaching my arms overhead.

My therapies helped me perform activities of daily living with these precautions in mind. In some physical therapy sessions, my therapist Kathryn would have me work on getting in and out of a car. In occupational therapy, we focused on negotiating getting in and out of a chair and a couch—hard to do when you can't use your arms! We also worked on performing simple household tasks such as loading and unloading a dishwasher, getting things in and out of the refrigerator, and doing laundry. I was amazed at the number of occupational tools available to help with these tasks, such as extendable reaching tools and dressing aids.

Sunnyview also provided social activities at night, such as Bingo or card games. I usually did not go to these as Keith faithfully visited me every night on his home from work, which luckily was close by. Crafting sessions were also offered, but to say I am not crafty is an understatement. I thought back to my craft session making rosary beads with Mrs. Sloan's third grade class whenever I saw a craft event notice. We were stringing beads for one student, Kristen, and the rope broke loose. Beads everywhere. The other assistant, Mrs. Whitcher, and I did our best to collect the beads. We came up two short. Mrs. Whitcher actually took beads off her necklace to complete the rosary. It was put together on a wing and a prayer. At Mass the next day, when Father Jim blessed the rosaries, I gulped when he picked up Kristen's. I saw Mrs. Sloan mouth to the student sitting next to her, "Be ready should the beads start to roll." Thank goodness nothing happened. I avoid crafts like the plague.

I did attend one activity—the visits from the therapy dogs Blue and Buttercup. They did not go room to room, but visited with patients in one of the activity rooms. I felt bittersweet after their first visit because I think it brought home how much I missed my dog Kovu. Just like Kovu, these dogs were loving and life affirming.

They came right up to my feet to be petted and would just lay there for a few minutes. They also seemed to have an attachment to Keith—I think that maybe they caught Kovu's scent. Unlike Kovu, they were relatively quiet and low key. Kovu's breed, the Keeshond, is recommended for therapy dog training, but I think you would need therapy after a session with him!

One skill I had to perform before being eligible for discharge was to go down and up a flight of stairs. I was nervous, since I had only gone up about six steps until that point. Kathryn assured me I was ready, so off to the stairwell we went. I knew she was right behind me if I needed her. Entering the stairwell, I was greeted with intense heat—the stairwells are not air-conditioned. "Let's do this," I said and began my trek down the steps, the relatively easy part. Kathryn let me know that I could take a break anytime I needed one. I made it down; now it was time to climb back up, the most challenging part. I took a drink of water, and began my ascent up the stairs. It took me over five minutes, but I did it! I was never so happy as to get back into my wheelchair in the air-conditioned hall.

In a little over a week, I had mastered what I needed to in both physical and occupational therapies. What kept me at Sunnyview so long were medical issues. My heart rate and blood pressure were erratic and my oxygen saturation remained low. I still had a large amount of fluid in my lungs, which is not uncommon in open-heart surgery patients.

I had two thoracentesis procedures—a somewhat painful procedure in which a long needle is inserted into the lung sac to remove fluid. Humor helps in these situations. I was very anxious about the first one, having no idea what to expect. Fortunately, the procedure could be done right in my room. A few nurses and a nursing student came in to assist the doctor. I had to sit on my bed and lean over my bedside table. I was given a local anesthetic, which actually turned out to be the most painful part of the procedure. One of my favorite nurses, Marian, held my hand. I was then ready for the needle to draw out the fluid.

"Thank goodness I can't see this," I mused. "I hate needles."

"Well it's a good thing you can't see this one, it's huge!" exclaimed the student nurse. We all saw Marian, who was still holding my hand, shoot her a glaring look. We all started to laugh.

Fortunately, the second procedure a week or so later went much better. At one point, leaning over the table while Dr. Michele Gorla was drawing out the fluid, I told the nurse, "I really want to be sitting out on my deck with a nice glass of Chardonnay."

"I'm pouring Rosé back here," chimed Dr. Gorla. I felt so comfortable with him; I asked if his practice would accept me as a patient after discharge. He is now my pulmonologist.

Something I really missed while at MGH and Sunnyview was fresh air. I had experienced it a bit when they wheeled me out from MGH to the ambulance and from the ambulance into Sunnyview. It had been heavenly. Nothing like a gorgeous bright blue sky and a soft breeze to lift your spirits. I had felt like an escapee. It left me wanting more! A little over a week into my stay at Sunnyview, I longingly looked outside the window of the fitness room and wistfully remarked to Kathryn that it was a gorgeous day. "C'mon," said Kathryn, "let's get you outside."

I couldn't yet walk too far, so Kathryn wheeled me down to the first floor and outdoors we went. We made two trips around the circular walkway in front of the entrance, and then sat on a bench until my "session" was over. I could have stayed there for hours!

All in all, I was beginning to feel like I was jinxed. It seemed every time the case manager came in to tell me I was being discharged, some new health issue would keep me there. The last straw was the nosebleed from hell. I was told on a Thursday that I would be going home that Saturday. Finally! Well, while in the bathroom Friday, my nose started to bleed, or should I say gush. My blood pressure must have climbed sky high since I cannot stand the sight of blood. Truth be told, I can't even walk by a blood drive without feeling queasy. It was horrendous—blood was pouring out of my nose and my mouth. It would stop, and then start up again. Somewhat ironic—my daily blood tests left me looking like a pincushion and here I was spouting blood like a geyser. After six hours of this, they brought me to the Ellis Hospital ER. Thank goodness, my husband met me there—he had been on his way to visit me when they carted me off. I was scared, anxious, and tired—not a good combination. The ER doctor was wonderful—from my hometown of Boston even. His Irish wit and easy-going attitude made me relax as much as I could. He believed the culprit was the blood thinner I was taking together with the relatively high level of oxygen I was on. He packed my nose and sent me back to Sunnyview with a full-face oxygen mask, since I couldn't use the normal cannula, and the positive thought that I might still be discharged the next day as planned.

Alas, that was not to happen. The Sunnyview team decided I needed to stay there to make sure there was no additional bleeding. I was so discouraged and depressed. What really ticked me off was when the case manager, with a big smile on her face, told me to stay positive and not complain. I had been positive and upbeat for two incredibly long weeks already. I had been the essence of upbeat. I was the poster child for positivity. C'mon! I wanted to give her piece of my mind, but it was too much effort.

I had always been excited about my therapy sessions and tried to improve each day. I also found out I was one of the staff favorites—one nurse told me every nurse wanted me as their patient when the manager made the daily assignments. My job was to make the best of my time at Sunnyview and work my hardest. I figured I was entitled to my five-minute pity party after the nosebleed nightmare.

The next four days were the longest in my life. I could do nothing—no physical therapy, no occupational therapy—nothing, for fear that the bleeding would begin again. All I could do was move from my bed to the chair and watch TV. Even reading was difficult. Because of the notorious "pumphead," I couldn't concentrate on the words. Postperfusion syndrome, also known as "pumphead" is an impairment of cognitive symptoms attributed to open heart surgery. Symptoms of postperfusion syndrome are subtle and can include decreased attention span, concentration difficulties, short-term memory loss, and decreased speeds of mental and motor responses.[8] Keith even brought me large print books but that didn't help me concentrate any better. With my packed nose, it was very hard to swallow, so eating and drinking were extremely difficult. My dear friend Carolyn came by with cannoli—she had a look of horror when she saw me! Carolyn had visited me the first week, and I had looked much better then. I also kept spitting and coughing up blood from all I had swallowed. I was tethered to a special oxygen set-up because of my post-nosebleed oxygen mask, so I couldn't even go back to visit with the therapy dogs Buttercup and Blue, who had so uplifted my spirits on their prior visits. This was brutal!

Finally, the day came to remove the packing. I was anxious about it, not only because of the envisioned pain but also for the likelihood of further bleeding. The case manager came in to remove it, and before I knew it, the packing was out. Whew! No sign of bleeding, thank goodness!

One further hurdle remained before I could be discharged. I felt like I was in a reality show—"To move on to the next level, you must..." I use a CPAP machine since I was diagnosed with sleep apnea a few years back. I needed to spend five hours on the CPAP at night before I could be discharged. This was to ensure that the CPAP would not trigger additional bleeding. Ah, but therein lies the rub—the respiratory therapist wanted me to use a full nose/mouth mask instead of my own nose mask to reduce the likelihood of a nosebleed. He did have a mask for me, but it wasn't a perfect fit. At that point, I would have eaten worms to get out of there—I could certainly endure five hours with an ill-fitting mask. It was hard to sleep with the mask, and I did not have a restful night. I had to sleep on my back, so I couldn't even toss and turn to get more comfortable. My five hours were up at 4 a.m. Promptly at 4:01, I rang for the nurse and asked her to take the contraption off me. When she did, she discovered a huge bruise on my forehead from the mask. No wonder I had a headache. I told her I needed my ticket punched and that she needed to note on my chart that I had lasted the five hours. Hurray!

On Thursday, July 23, the case manager came in and said I would be going home the following Monday or Tuesday. "Please," I begged, "move every mountain you have to and get me out of here Monday. I don't want to risk anything else happening!" She agreed on Monday. I would be heading home in four days! I said every prayer I knew asking for continued health and no other "event" occurrence. My friend Carolyn's mother had sent me some prayers for healing which I prayed fervently.

I knew my time at Sunnyview was coming to an end when I had to redo the initial benchmark test. This served as a tangible measure of my progress. I managed to walk around the entire floor! Quite an improvement from the initial test. I was ready to go home. Another task I had to accomplish before I could be discharged was to show evidence that I could manage my medications myself. I just chuckled at this, since I had managed not only my medications, but also my mom's and my dad's when they were living with us. The nurse gave me my medications schedule. At the appropriate time, I was to ring for the medications nurse. This didn't even last the day. That afternoon, the medications nurse smiled at me saying, "You got this; you're good to go."

While my stay at Sunnyview was longer than I would have liked and sometimes difficult, I did meet many wonderful people, including my physical therapist, Kathryn. We hit it off from the start, and I truly enjoyed our sessions. I worked my butt off, but it gave me a sense of accomplishment and strength. She was like my cheerleader—Kathryn told me that at every patient progress meeting she informed the team that medical issues were holding me back, not physical. Eventually, I even wore out things to do with the occupational therapists—how many times can you put dishes in and out of the dishwasher? God bless them for thinking up new and innovative things to keep me occupied. I particularly enjoyed my visits to the hospital gift shops with the occupational therapist. I was becoming a force to contend with maneuvering that walker in the store—hey, a girl's gotta shop! I wished I'd had my charge card!

My nurse Ryan would constantly cheer me up, telling me I would eventually get back to my old self, which truly did not seem possible. When I visited the hospital four months after discharge—sans walker and oxygen—he gave me a big hug, telling me "I knew you would do it." Like at MGH, all the nurses and support staff were caring, compassionate, and brightened my days. One aide would stop in every afternoon and remind me to watch *The Ellen DeGeneres Show* to make sure I had my daily dose of laughter.

I was also blessed to have a wonderful roommate, Lois. She was a delightful elderly woman with an upbeat, positive attitude. Her daughter and son-in-law were ministers, and one Sunday when they came to visit, Keith and I joined them in an impromptu prayer/communion service. Whenever two or more are gathered in His name—it was one of the most moving faith experiences I have ever had. We thanked God for the healing that had taken place and asked for future healing. We prayed for our own and our family members' strength in dealing with our situations. I felt a shift in my perception and knew I would make it through to complete recovery, which I sometimes had doubted.

The nurses would love to stop by our room when our families were visiting. We always had our share of laughter and good conversation. It even led to my own Edie-inspired bathroom moment. We were talking about fun things to do in the area over the summer, and the popular Saratoga Race Course—a thoroughbred horse racing track in Saratoga Springs—came up. I was taking many diuretics, and when I had to go, I really had to move quickly. "Bathroom break," I chimed. Getting me out of the bed (difficult with sternal precautions), hooking me up to a portable oxygen tank, and getting my walker took the nurse time. I didn't think I would make it. In the spirit of things, when I made it to the bathroom door I exclaimed, "And Lasix Running is rounding the last turn for the finish." We all roared so loud everyone in the hall stuck his or her head in to see what was going on.

Finally, discharge day arrived. It was June 26, a little over five weeks from my surgery. So much for my plan of being home by Memorial Day! I was longing to see home and my furry friend Kovu. I told Keith he had better come early before anything else could happen. One of the aides came in to pack for me and get my things "organized." I now know why many women are in charge of packing for family vacations—some men are packing challenged! I wasn't going to complain—I was going home!

Keith arrived with my friend Pam. I was glad to see her; I knew I wouldn't remember all the discharge orders and Keith was already overwhelmed. Since Pam was a former cardiac nurse, she would know what questions to ask and would be a valuable resource. She accompanied us home to help get me into the house with my walker and oxygen tank in tow, since those tasks were difficult for Keith to manage.

I was ecstatic when I walked out of Sunnyview and went into my car. I felt like a kid on the last day of school. Walking into my house was like returning to my childhood home—it was familiar, yet unfamiliar at the same time. Everything seemed in place, though there were small changes: a pillow moved to another chair, a vase placed in a new spot. It felt strange knowing that life had gone on in this house without me. By this point, I was starving and craving a sub. Keith went to our local favorite sub shop and got us lunch. My first meal at home! That was the best darn veggie sub ever!

The Real Recovery Begins—A Series of Firsts

The first days at home were difficult. While I was giddy with happiness to be home, I was somewhat hesitant—what do I do now? At Sunnyview, my day was pretty much planned and organized for me. Now it was up to me. Everything at first was a struggle. How can I get myself into the kitchen chair, how can I maneuver my way into the bathroom? Because I was still under sternal precautions, getting in and out of the kitchen chair took a herculean effort. Keith would have to pull the chair out for me, pull the table towards me, and make adjustments as needed. Keith was also just figuring out how he could best help me since we were venturing in unknown territory. I had to get used to negotiating my home with a walker, getting on and off the couch, and taking bowl baths. I was still on oxygen, so the length of the tubing limited my movement.

Thank goodness, Keith had some personal time available. He was able to stay home with me for about a week and a half. During this time, we worked out all the kinks and created a daily routine. This included having things such as clothing, towels, and food readily available and accessible. My new armoire was the love seat in the living room where Keith stacked my clothing and towels in neat piles. Luckily, I was entitled to a few at-home physical and occupational therapist visits. They showed me how to maneuver myself into the kitchen chair and how to sidestep my way with the walker into the bathroom. They encouraged me to try climbing a small number of stairs each day. I was hesitant to try this alone, so I always made sure Keith was around to assist if necessary.

I slept in our family room in a reclining chair and Keith slept nearby on the couch. I use the word "sleep" here loosely. I would only doze off for a while and then wake up in a pool of sweat. Night sweats, I found out later, are common after cardiac surgery. Should you experience these, check your temperature to make sure you do not have a fever. If your temperature is 101 degrees Fahrenheit or greater, call your doctor. Otherwise, make yourself as comfortable as possible by changing linens/coverings and bed clothes. I know Keith was as sleep deprived as I was during this time. We tried many configurations of sheets and blankets to limit this sweatiness and subsequent chills, which eventually went away.

While I never experienced sharp pain at the incision, I often felt a heaviness or pulling there, almost as if someone was moving a brick across my chest. This generally occurred in the morning. I had painkillers but did not want to rely on them too much. Eventually, I was able to drop down from a dose in the morning and evening to just using acetaminophen.

Thank goodness it was summer, since I could live in loose and comfortable clothing. Even though I had lost the additional surgery weight and then some, I discovered I could not wear my regular bras because they aggravated my incision. I wanted some support, and discovered that Fruit of the Loom sports bras worked best for me. The hospital did provide me with some bras post-surgery, but they were not comfortable. I sometimes needed to put gauze inside the hospital-provided bras to keep the bra from rubbing against the incision. To avoid retaining fluid, I also wore compression socks—quite a fashion statement with shorts, to be sure!

I think my initial recovery period was as hard for Keith as it was for me. He had to help me with simple tasks, such as dressing, getting to the table, bathing, all of which seemed to take twice as long. I did not want Keith to experience caregiver burnout. If you are concerned about caregiver stress, check what local resources are available. Most areas have some organizations (e.g. Community Caregivers) that provide caregiver support as well as services for the patient, such as transportation. Make sure your caregiver takes time to rest and rejuvenate. I encouraged Keith to make time for his favorite activities, guitar playing and gardening. We tried to keep things as easy as possible, such as preparing only simple meals and using paper plates. We didn't even bother opening our pool since it would require a lot of upkeep. Let your caregiver know he needs to take care of his needs—he will be better prepared to care for you. Ask for help from friends. They often want to help but just need some direction as to what you need. During this time, we discovered the grocery delivery service that many supermarkets now offer. It proved to be a great time saver.

Friends and neighbors may want to visit you once you are home and settled. At first, you will want to set limits on the visit length. For me, I found 20 minutes was about all I could handle the first few weeks at home because of fatigue. Your caregiver can enforce these limits if you feel uncomfortable doing so.

Cardiac surgery patients sometimes experience depression. Emotionally, I had good days and bad, but I never experienced a long-term depression. I found having a daily schedule really helped me, as did keeping track of my recovery progress. Depression can be very difficult for the caregiver as well, since the patient may show lack of appreciation and cooperation. Signs of depression include difficulties thinking and concentrating, spontaneous crying spells, and feelings of hopelessness or thoughts of death or suicide. Caregivers, be sure to get extra help and a professional involved should your loved one exhibit symptoms of depression.

One lesson I continue to learn from recovery is to appreciate the simple things in life and not take anything for granted. Life for me became a series of firsts. More often than not, they were just a series of first steps leading to the ability to accomplish an entire task.

Keith eventually had to go back to work. I remember the first day I was "home alone." Although I was still under sternal precautions, I thought I could manage by myself. I just asked Keith to leave things that I might need out on the counter so I would not have to reach for them. I suddenly felt free and almost "normal." I found that I needed to always get dressed and make a daily schedule of sorts so I did not feel like a patient. I still could not drive so I was stuck in the house. Even though I needed a walker and oxygen I could feel myself getting stronger, but I was not yet well enough to venture outdoors. Since the steps from our house leading to the backyard and deck do not have a railing, I did not feel comfortable using them. I found enough things to do—email friends, read, listen to music, watch TV, or even just watch the birds at the feeder. So much for my plan of enjoying summer walks and sitting on my deck!

The first time I cooked a meal I planned a very simple chicken marsala. Keith purchased the necessary ingredients the night before and left out the bakeware since I couldn't yet reach it. I was starting to feel more like a household contributor, not a patient. It felt good to be cooking again and taking some of the stress of meal preparation off Keith. That was the best chicken marsala I had had in a long time!

The first time I did laundry after three weeks home (darn, I probably should have milked this one more), I could just start the washer and fold clean clothes. Within a few more weeks, I was able to load and unload both the washer and dryer.

Another first was going out for breakfast at our favorite diner, which Keith and I frequently enjoyed pre-surgery. Our last breakfast there had been on our way up to Boston for the surgery. Keith hadn't gone there after returning home from Boston. He just didn't feel like going without me. Getting me ready to go out was almost as bad as getting kids out the door—did I have my walker, did I have my pillow to place under the seat belt to protect my chest, did I have an extra oxygen tank? It was an effort, but well worth it—our former routines were slowly but surely returning. We even made it out to dinner with some friends, oxygen tank and reserve in tow.

Walking at home was a strategic exercise. Wherever I walked, Keith and I had to plan it out first. We always had a chair at hand for me to sit in if I became tired. My first time walking without a walker was somewhat scary, but I could feel myself get stronger each day. Even this occurred in stages—I first walked alone during the day, using the walker only if I got up in the middle of the night. By August, I was walking solo 24/7! I was starting to feel more like my old self.

I remember the first time I walked upstairs and took a shower. I had been limited to bowl baths downstairs, which were OK, but not great. Even these took quite a bit of planning to have wash and rinse water available and to avoid getting chilled. I needed some sort of reinforcement bar in the shower, even though we had purchased a shower chair. We went back and forth about having a bar professionally installed or just finding one ourselves. After some research, we purchased Moen 12-Inch Suction Balance Assist Bath Grip, which was relatively inexpensive at $15 and works just fine. It has the advantage of being portable. Keith wanted to make sure I was strong enough to venture upstairs, since with his disability he would not be much help should I have difficulty. We did several test walks, with me going partway up the stairs and then back down. I would pause at each step and assess if I could go on. We planned each walk and stuck to the plan each time. Also, all this time I was tethered to my oxygen concentrator and had to navigate carefully with the oxygen tubing so I wouldn't trip. Then, on the day of lift off, Keith positioned a chair at the top of the stairs just in case. With plenty of oxygen tubing, I made the climb. All ten feet of it. It took almost five minutes. Edmund Hillary at the top of Mt. Everest couldn't have felt better. Then, on to the shower. Keith positioned the shower chair in the shower and got the water running to the correct temperature. Even with the grab bar, I did not feel comfortable enough standing up to retrieve soap and shampoo from the shower caddy. Keith handed them to me when I was ready. Ahhhh! I felt like I was in heaven—warm water cascading over me, being able to use my favorite body wash—pure bliss!

Finally, I got the OK to drive. It was so good not to have to rely on Keith, Colin, or my friend Pam to take me places. I felt so free being able to run to the market to pick up some groceries or go to the library. I started out slowly, just driving locally.

Another huge milestone was being able to get physically active again and participate in my favorite activities. I couldn't wait to start cardiac rehab. At my first post-surgery visit with Dr. Dibble, he didn't think I was ready. About a month later, on August 7, I had a telehealth video call with Dr. Bhatt in Boston. She thought I was ready, and proceeded to text Dr. Dibble to confer with him. He texted back, from the beach while on vacation, saying I was good to go! The wonders of technology! And the benefits of having doctors who work well together! Within a few weeks, I enrolled in a great cardiac rehab program at St. Peter's Cardiac Rehabilitation and Wellness.

I was thrilled, albeit a little scared, at my first cardiac rehab session on September 1. Pam offered to bring me since I did not yet feel comfortable driving, even though Dr. Dibble had given me the OK. The exit off the highway involved a lot of head turning to see adequately, which could have aggravated my incision.

The notion of 36 sessions seemed overwhelming at first. To help keep me motivated and focused, I set a goal of completing the sessions before my December appointment with Dr. Bhatt. I began the program while I was still on oxygen, and it was not fun lugging that tank around. At the initial six-minute walk test, I almost tripped over the tank and myself!

I'll always remember my first outdoor walk alone. I had been feeling somewhat down over the summer since I had not felt well enough to walk outdoors. Not only was I dealing with the walker for a good part of the summer, but also I just did not have the strength. However, after a few weeks at cardiac rehab I felt strong enough to venture out alone without the walker. I now had a small portable oxygen tank, which was cumbersome but easier to lug than the large tank. It was a glorious September day, with the leaves almost at the peak of color. How invigorating it was to be out in the brilliant sun on this perfect day!

Experiencing these firsts helped me recognize how far I had truly come since May. I often felt disappointed at the pace of my recovery, but then I'd review my progress and see the significant strides I'd made. It's amazing how many simple everyday things in life we take for granted until we can't do them. Experiencing these things anew brought back a childlike joy and wonder. Even by September, I still had a recovery journey ahead of me, with several firsts I hoped to achieve, such as getting rid of the oxygen tank, walking my furry friend Kovu, and getting into the pool in the YMCA. I knew they would happen all in good time.

Let the Doctor Visits Begin

During the first few months of recovery, I spent most of my days going to doctors' appointments. Until I was able to drive myself, Keith or my son needed to take me. It seemed to take so long to get out of the house—depending on where we were going, I needed a transport chair and extra oxygen tanks. Just getting me into the offices was an event. Let me not forget the simple joys of getting my walker onto an elevator without getting stuck while Keith dragged the oxygen tank along.

At least once a week, I visited one of my friendly phlebotomists, Melissa or Michin, for a Coumadin (blood thinner) check. I felt like I was in a Cheers spinoff—everybody knew my name and just ushered me right in. Thank goodness, they used a finger stick so I did not have to get the full blood draw. My levels were up and down, hence the many visits. Of course, just when we got it regulated, I was taken off Coumadin so I no longer required the finger sticks.

Most of my appointments were local, but eventually in July it was time for me to return to MGH for my post-surgery visit. I felt very anxious about this; I did not believe I was progressing fast enough. I was also dreading the long trip. I was just thankful it wasn't wintertime.

Dr. MacGillivray was thrilled with my progress. He immediately noted that my color was great and I had no edema. I thought at first he was kidding. I was still using a walker and wheelchair, had a tank of oxygen, and felt discouraged. "Just give it time," he told me. I wanted a date, timeframe, details—there were none, just the recognition that I would be improving every day. Every congenital surgery is different and so is the recovery. It had been too much of a bumpy ride for me, but he encouraged me to stay positive. When he told me my recovery time would be "exponential," I just gave him a blank stare. I could not even envision being back to my former self.

After my appointment, Dr. Bhatt came up to greet me. She also thought I looked good. When I complained that recovery was slower than I anticipated, she noted that I had undergone the most difficult surgery from which to recover. Good thing she didn't tell me this beforehand! My heart had been pretty much "remade," so much so that Keith now jokingly referred to me as "Deb 2.0." Dr. MacGillivray laughed appreciatively when Keith told him my new nickname.

Thank goodness I have a sense of humor. On our way home from Boston, we stopped along the Mass Pike for lunch. Poor Keith—it took him forever to lug out the oxygen tank and get the transport chair set up. At this point, I was still not comfortable walking long distances, even with the walker. The path to the entrance was not only rough, but also had an almost imperceptible slope. I thought Keith had the chair and was moving me along faster than usual; he thought I was "driving." But in reality, the chair was running its own race.

"Please stop that chair!" Keith called out.

"Woman on the loose," I warned, and thank goodness a big burly gentleman stopped me and the chair from what would have been a very nasty entrance into the rest area.

Most weeks I had two or three doctors' appointments, but by the end of August, I was driving myself to them. By October, I seemed to be at a standstill. I was still on oxygen full-time and didn't think I would ever get off it. Therefore, it was with much trepidation that I went for my checkup with Dr. Gorla, my pulmonologist. He had performed another thoracentesis after my first post-surgery visit with him. I was hoping that by now my lungs were clear. He listened to my lungs and said they sounded good and this was confirmed when he read the x-ray—no fluid and no scarring! He asked how I was doing and I expressed my frustration with still being on oxygen. Since my oxygen saturation was at a reasonable level, he had me do a six-minute test, during which I walked back and forth down the corridor. A nurse monitored my oxygen saturation levels. I tried not to look, but couldn't help noticing that my levels were going up and down the whole time. I just tried to focus on my breathing to ensure my lungs were getting sufficient oxygen. Near the end of the test, the nurse went into the doctor's office—I figured I was doomed. I was wrong! I could now be off oxygen, except for cardiac rehab and at night. I was thrilled. While I recognize the oxygen was life supporting, it often seemed like an albatross as it prohibited me from many activities I enjoyed.

For many years before surgery, my ankles and calves were swollen. Dr. Gorla asked how the swelling in my ankles was. "Look," I exclaimed, wiggling my sandaled feet, "I have ankles—no swelling!" It was a milestone for me—my feet no longer looked like inflated latex gloves.

Since Dr. Gorla's office is attached to Sunnyview, I decided to stop in after my appointment. Heck, I didn't have to lug around the oxygen! It was great to see my former therapists, nurses, and caretakers, especially Kathryn. I felt like a kid coming home with a straight A report card. They were thrilled with the progress I had made, and I welcomed the opportunity to thank them in person.

No oxygen during the day meant I could now go swimming. I could not wait for my first visit to the YMCA pool. I wanted to capture the moment, so I took my cell phone to take a picture. The aquatics coordinator Cindy came over as soon as she saw me— she was delighted to see me back. I asked her if she wouldn't mind taking a photo of me. Luckily, the pool wasn't crowded, so we wouldn't be disturbing anyone. When I looked at the picture of me right after surgery with the tubes and machines around me, and then the picture of me swimming in the pool, I realized how far I had come in just five months!

My annual checkup with Dr. Bhatt was in December. Back to MGH we went—a much easier trip than in July! She was pleased with my progress and thought I looked great. When she asked about cardiac rehab, I told her I met my goal of completing the 36 sessions before our appointment. She was thrilled.

Since we had arrived in Boston the night before my appointment, Keith and I were able to meet Marcy and Ben for dinner at one of my favorite seafood restaurants. I hadn't seen them since they visited me at MGH. We had a joyous holiday celebration!

Lessons Learned

One lesson learned in my interactions with my medical team is that you truly need to be an active participant in and advocate for your own health care. You can't wait for doctors to tell you what you are capable of doing. You have to ask. At my appointment with Dr. Dibble in August, I asked him if I could drive. Dr. Dibble seemed surprised that I asked and said sure, as though I could have been driving for weeks! I should have asked him earlier!

Sometimes rather crazy things happen. When I left Sunnyview, my "orders" included visiting my primary care physician. In fact, Sunnyview had scheduled the appointment for me. The appointment was with a physician's assistant, not my primary care doctor. He asked me what I was doing there, and I replied, "You tell me!" We both had a good laugh. He said there wasn't much he could do for me at that point, so he updated my medications list and home I went. I wished I had checked before the appointment to see if it was necessary—I might have saved Keith and me the trip.

You are your own best health care advocate. If you can't seem to build a relationship with your doctor, change to another one. Several years before surgery, I just wasn't happy with my primary care doctor. He was certainly qualified, but I didn't feel comfortable with him. I switched to another physician and she is wonderful! I was truly amazed at all the insurance hoops I had to go through to make this change, but it was worth it. I also ended up having to find a new endocrinologist. I had been seeing a physician's assistant at a relatively large practice. I had not returned in over a year due to dealing with my ill parents, both of whom had moved in with my family. When I called to reschedule, the secretary informed me that the practice had "released" me. I found another endocrinologist, Dr. Sara Clark, who is just fantastic. She recognizes the complexities in my care and thinks outside the box. My first appointment with her lasted over an hour. She asked me all sorts of questions, such as how was I sleeping, could I lose weight easily, was I often fatigued. She suggested I get tested for sleep apnea, which it turns out I have. Without her big picture view, it might not have been diagnosed. I felt like a number in the other practice—in and out in 10 minutes. Here, I am a person. I wished I had sent my former endocrinologist a thank you note!

As the captain of your health care team, you need to make sure that you are doing all you can to stay healthy. Eating right, getting enough sleep, exercising—these are not luxuries. Also as the captain, you have the right and responsibility to question your doctors and change providers if necessary.

The Journey Continues

Many congenital heart patients and their families have the misconception that surgery "cures" congenital heart disease. It does not. While surgery can temporarily address the condition, it cannot cure it. That's why it is important for all adult congenital heart patients, even if they seem asymptomatic, to receive lifelong care at a center specializing in treating adults with CHD. The Adult Congenital Heart Association website, achaheart.org, has a list of adult congenital heart clinics.

While there are guidelines for recovery, they are just that. No matter how long and hopeless the process seems, trust that you will get better. My first day at cardiac rehab, I could walk only 700 feet and my machine settings were all at the lowest resistance. On one machine, the resistance had been inadvertently set at seven instead of one, and I couldn't budge it. On "graduation day," I walked 1500 feet, was not on oxygen, and the level seven setting on the machine was a breeze. And by this time, I was driving myself to cardiac rehab.

I learned to take recovery one day at a time. Some days seemed longer than others did, to be sure. When I started to feel discouraged with my progress, I just thought back to where I had been the prior week, the prior month, the prior two months, etc. Have someone take a picture of you immediately post-surgery and then take some pictures during the recovery process. The camera doesn't lie—you will have a nice visual record of how far you have come. Celebrate each small success, no matter how insignificant it may seem. Recognizing these victories will motivate you and help you along your recovery journey. Keith always brought home a beautiful floral bouquet to celebrate my milestones.

One surprising post-surgery transformation I experienced was having my finger nails grow longer and stronger! I had experienced "spoon nails" and brittle nails before surgery. They cracked and broke easily. My nails now grow long enough for me to splurge on an occasional manicure!

How far I had come became crystal clear when I saw my endocrinologist, Dr. Clark, in early October. At this point, I was still tethered to my oxygen tank. She told me I looked fantastic and then asked me why I had oxygen. When I told her about my surgery, her eyes opened wide in surprise and she remarked, "I would have had no idea that you had been through something like that except for the oxygen." Sometimes other people's lenses are clearer than yours are.

You need to learn to put yourself first during recovery. This is hard, especially for women who are so used to putting family and others first. This may mean learning to say "no." Maybe this is not the year for you to hold that Memorial Day picnic or host the Christmas cookie exchange. If people don't understand, it's their problem, not yours.

You may decide to make some life changes based on your recovery and newfound appreciation for life. I have come to realize that life is too short and have made some major life changes. In the fall of 2016, I retired from teaching. Although I may eventually substitute teach from time to time, I find more satisfaction and reward in focusing on women's and congenital heart-health issues, be it through speaking, writing, or volunteering.

Make sure you are eating healthfully and exercising at your level. For many cardiac patients, developing and maintaining an exercise routine can be daunting. A good cardiac rehab program is a blessing. You will be monitored and will come to know what your exercise boundaries are. After completing the monitoring phase of the program, you can often continue in their regular exercise or wellness program. If you are on your own, you need to develop an action plan that works for you. It doesn't have to be cast in stone, but it needs to be something you can track and assess. Here's where SMART goals come into play. Your goals need to be Specific, Measurable, Attainable, Relevant, and Time bound.[9] A SMART goal is tailor made for you and by you, reflecting your personal preferences and lifestyle. When you identify your most important goals, you can begin to figure out ways to succeed. You develop the attitudes, abilities, skills, and financial capacity to reach them. I fully realize that my goals and their related action plans will probably need to be recast from time to time depending on my health situation.

My trainer at the YMCA once told me that people with a fitness "event" goal (such as walking a 5K) tend to stay with a fitness program longer than those who do not have a goal. Being a "high achiever" type, I need both long-term and short-term goals to keep me motivated. With that in mind, I set a short- term goal of walking a 5K as close to the one-year anniversary date of my surgery as possible.

I have completed three so far, and all were memorable experiences. The first was the Mother Lovin' 5K, held about 45 minutes away in Saratoga Springs, NY on Mother's Day, 2016—less than a year after my surgery. Rain was in the forecast, but my favorite TV weatherman, Bob Kovachick, assured us it would stop by 9:15 a.m., precisely the time the race started. I woke up Mother's Day and looked out the window. Not a drip, not a drop, but a deluge. I looked at Keith; he looked back at me and said, "If you don't go, and it clears up, you'll be kicking yourself." I decided to take the plunge. If it was really bad, I could decide not to walk. We were quiet the entire ride up; all you could hear were the sheets of rain pelting the car.

At about 9:00 a.m. the rain turned to drizzle. I decided to go for it. I started out with the crowd, but soon I was walking alone. I just kept going. Thankfully, there were race monitors to show me the way, since not another walker or runner was in sight. Finally, I came to the last race monitor, who exclaimed, "You're almost there—the finish is just over these two hills!"

"Oh hell no," I said, "not hills, I can't do hills, especially at the end of the race."

The race monitor, with his dog, offered to walk with me since I was obviously the last finisher. He kept saying, "We're almost there."

And I kept responding, "You said that 15 minutes ago."

Even the police assigned to the race left before I finished. In fact, they gave me the "thumbs up" from their patrol car as they passed me on the course. Another car came by. It was Keith and the race director making sure I was OK. I had gone past the estimated finish time I had given Keith and he was worried. I had not factored in the darn hills. They offered to drive me back, and when the race monitor said, "You're almost there!" I couldn't help but laugh. Yes, I finished and yes, I was dead last—but I did it.

The 5K I had been anxiously awaiting was the Freihofer's Run for Women, scheduled for June 4, 2016. I had attempted this race about 15 years ago but did not finish. It has been run for 38 years, and brings elite and amateur runners together. Usually over 3,000 runners/walkers compete. My friend Carolyn offered to walk with me. I was slow, it was hot, but we finished! I was dead last again, but greatly appreciated the clapping from the crowd when the race announcer's voice boomed out, "Here comes our last place finisher; quite an accomplishment to stick it out in this heat." One more thing to cross off my bucket list.

I learned a great deal from my third 5K, the Corelle 5K, held in Corning, NY on October 1, 2016. We arrived the night before the race, since Corning is a four-hour drive, but we should have arrived two nights before to become better acclimated to our surroundings. To say I did not sleep well would be an understatement. In addition, the mini muffin I had for breakfast on race day was not enough. Due to little sleep and insufficient nutrition, this became my most difficult 5K walk to date. However, I did finish the race! I felt like a movie star as I crossed the finish line! Several photographers were taking my picture and the small crowd cheered for me. I was truly humbled by and appreciative of the volunteers who walked the last mile with me and hugged me at the finish line—I could not have finished without their support and encouragement. They were a true blessing. I was elated to show off my medal at the "meet up" that afternoon with fellow racers from Coach Jenny's Challenge Facebook Group who were there to race in the half or full marathon the next day.

Also remember that emotionally, not just physically, you will have good days and bad. For me, a bad day usually followed a string of a few good days. In sensing this pattern, I came to realize that I had probably been stretching my boundaries a bit much and my body and mind just said "enough."

However, if you continually feel depressed or feel like you need additional help, seek out the support of a therapist. While I had only planned to see my therapist, Dr. Das, before surgery, I decided to continue a monthly session. I found I was experiencing anxiety over things that never bothered me before, such as being in a car or driving on the throughway. She has helped me feel more in charge of my life. Now, I just check in with her every few months or so if I feel the need.

I admit it—I'm a type A, "can do it all myself" type of gal. Recognizing my limitations and accepting help was very hard for me. I was used to being the caregiver, not the one that needed care. I learned to graciously accept help and support. If I needed a ride somewhere due to a conflict with Keith's schedule, I felt comfortable asking someone. During the Freihofer's 5K, I let Carolyn know that she could go ahead of me, but she didn't and I didn't insist. She stuck with me the entire way, and I am grateful. I now recognize that the person helping me benefits as much as I do. Ask for assistance when you need it and take the time to thank those who helped you in any way during your recovery. I'll never forget the prayer booklets and prayer cards Carolyn's mom sent to me while I was at Sunnyview. They provided much solace during some dark days and I made sure to thank her.

Surround yourself with positive people. Recovery is difficult enough without bringing in negativity. If you are holding on to a friendship that is trying, let it go. Seek out those who lift you up, not bring you down. Support groups can help. For me, Coach Jenny's Challenge Facebook Group was invaluable. I received encouragement and motivation that helped me stay positive during recovery. They cheered every step I took no matter how small. It was and continues to be a very positive environment—I never felt silly sharing my one block walk with these marathoners and triathletes. Several of them were facing issues as well, and seeing their posts encouraged me to press on. They also held me accountable—I knew someone would ask me what I did for exercise that day.

Give back. I remember feeling very alone and scared with my heart issues. In discussing weekend plans with a work colleague, I mentioned to her that I was going to Boston to see my cardiologist. She asked why, and I told her I had a rare congenital defect, Ebstein's Anomaly. She burst into tears, and through her tears told me her baby daughter was just diagnosed with the same condition. She said seeing me alive and well gave her hope. I decided then and there that I wanted to help others living with heart disease in some way. In seeking out help for myself, I came across two wonderful organizations that I am honored to volunteer with. As a Heart to Heart Ambassador with the Adult Congenital Heart Association, I provide peer-to-peer support by phone or email to others living with congenital heart disease. As a WomenHeart Champion with WomenHeart: The National Coalition for Women with Heart Disease, I give talks throughout New York and western Massachusetts to women about heart health and encourage them to live healthfully. I'm hoping in some small way that I can make a difference. I also receive support and encouragement from these organizations as well. I still get anxious before my doctors' appointments and have doubts about how my condition will progress in the future. Talking with others who have these same fears has helped me work through these issues by encouraging me to stay positive and to look at how far I have come.

Think and dream big. Don't set limits for yourself— you never know what you can accomplish until you try. I've discovered that I'm the only one that can set limits on myself, not my health care team. In a strange way, not knowing my limits has been freeing—I have no one telling me I can't accomplish something. As Henry Ford once said, "Whether you think you can or think you can't, you're right." Having a life full of optimism and expectation will keep you young and bring you joy.

Surround yourself with beauty. One of the nicest things my husband did was to put a bird feeder right outside the window near my recliner. There is something calming about just sitting and watching the birds come to feed. Listen to music. Light a candle.

Have faith that you will get better and can get back to a normal life, even if it is a new normal. Knowing that people were praying for me and wishing me well helped me on my journey. You can emerge from this experience stronger and more determined to live life fully. You will find the strength and motivation to pursue goals or dreams that you may have left dormant. After getting through this most difficult experience, I am courageously pursuing my dreams—writing this (and maybe another!) book, getting back to goal weight, and completing a half marathon.

Most of all, I recognize that each day is a gift. I find I now have a childlike awe and wonder about the world around me. Taking a simple walk through the woods has become almost spiritual. I used to complain about getting old, now I am grateful for each day I wake up. I don't worry about the "small stuff" anymore. Being thankful for life will help you live happily and healthfully. You can thrive, not just survive, with heart disease. You owe it to yourself!

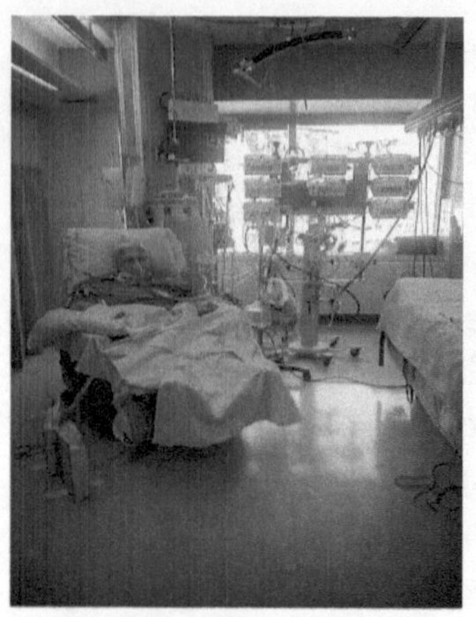

May 22, 2015
Post-surgery

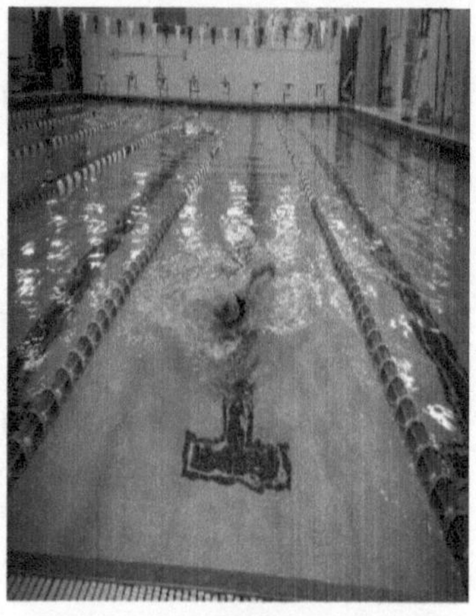

October 22, 2015
First swim at the
YMCA

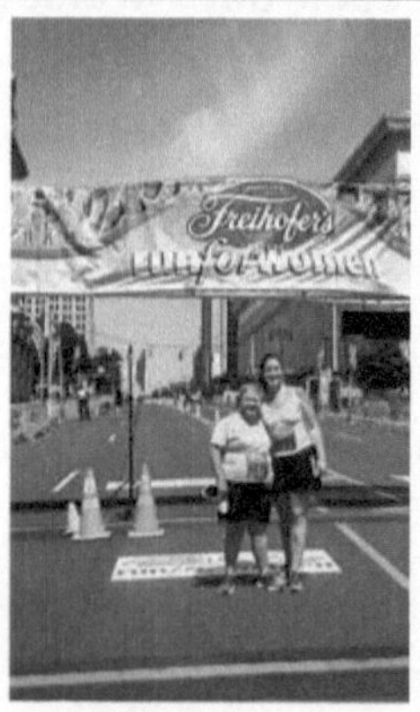

June 4, 2016
Finally a Freihofer's
finisher

References

1. http://www.cdc.gov/ncbddd/heartdefects/data.html

2. Silverman, Mark E. "A view from the millennium: the practice of cardiology circa 1950 and thereafter." Journal of the American College of Cardiology 33, no.4 (April 1999): 1141-1151

3. http://emedicine.medscape.com/article/903579-overview#a5

4. https://www.deltadentalins.com/oral_health/heart.html

5. https://consumer.healthday.com/senior-citizen-information-31/misc-death-and-dying-news-172/getting-teeth-pulled-before-heart-surgery-may-pose-serious-risks-685241.html

6. http://www.bostonmagazine.com/2006/05/these-doctors-will-see-you-now/

7. https://www.verywell.com/sternal-precautions-2696084

8. http://www.scientificamerican.com/article/pumphead-heart-lung-machine/

9. http://www.smart-goals-guide.com/smart-goal.html

Resources

I found the following resources helpful in dealing with heart disease and surgery:

Organizations

Adult Congenital Heart Association

(https://www.achaheart.org/). The mission of the Adult Congenital Heart Association (ACHA) is to improve and extend the lives of the millions born with heart defects through education, advocacy, and the promotion of research. The website provides a listing of adult congenital heart clinics, information on congenital heart defects, opportunities to receive support, and more.

American Heart Association

(http://www.heart.org/HEARTORG/). The mission of the American Heart Association is to build healthier lives free of cardiovascular diseases and stroke. The website provides tips on leading a heart-healthy lifestyle, information on heart-related conditions, resources for caregivers and educators, and more.

Mended Hearts

(http://mendedhearts.org). The mission of Mended Hearts is dedicated to inspiring hope and improving the quality of life for heart patients and their families through ongoing peer-to-peer support. Mended Hearts educates members on coping with heart disease. They educate family, friends, and loved ones about the facts of heart disease and what to expect during recovery.

WomenHeart: The National Coalition for Women with Heart Disease

(http://www.womenheart.org). WomenHeart's mission is to improve the health and quality of life of women living with or at risk of heart disease and to advocate for their benefit. Along with information about heart disease in women, WomenHeart offers support groups and provides speakers on heart disease.

Books

Huddleston, Peggy. *Prepare for Surgery, Heal Faster.* 1996, Cambridge: Angel River Press.

I used both the CDs and book to curb my pre-surgery anxiety and fears. It will help you prepare for any type of surgery, not just cardiac. The CDs really calmed me, and after listening to them, I was able to use some of the techniques to relax myself and remove some of the anxiety of the hospital stay and accompanying (sometimes invasive) procedures. The author also provides some useful information about setting up a support network to help you. Once home I continued listening to the relaxation CD and I was able to wean myself off prescription painkillers fairly quickly.

Lichtenberg, Maggie. *The Open Heart Companion: Preparation and Guidance for Open-Heart Surgery Recovery. 2006, Santa Fe: Open Heart Publishing.*

This beautifully written book balances telling a personal story with providing concrete information about all aspects of open heart surgery. Read this book well before surgery if possible. I found her checklists to be quite helpful.

Oz, Mehmet. *Healing from the Heart: How Unconventional Wisdom Unleashes the Power of Modern Medicine.* 1998, New York: Plume.

Although written some time ago, I found this book very helpful in illuminating the potential of complementary medicine. The book contains stories of patients Dr. Oz treated using these techniques. The emergence of Cardiac Wellness Centers in many hospitals points to the increasing acceptance and use of these techniques.

Pick, Adam. *The Patient's Guide to Heart Valve Surgery.* 2015, HeartValveSurgery.com.

This first-hand account takes you through all stages of the surgery process, from learning that you need surgery through recovering from surgery. I appreciated his honesty and discussion of the ups and downs of the recovery process.

Selkow, Warren and Selkow, Donna. *The Simplified Handbook for Living with Heart Disease and Other Chronic Diseases.* 2009, http://www.simplehand.org/.

This is another patient/caregiver collaboration. The authors offer much practical advice about living with heart disease and other chronic diseases. I found it engaging, often amusing, and thought provoking.

Sood, Amit. *The Mayo Clinic Guide to Stress-Free Living.* 2013, Boston: DeCapo.

Dealing with a congenital heart defect can be stressful. This book offers many wonderful suggestions for developing practices that will help reduce stress.

Wallack, Mark M.D. and Colby, Jane. *Back to Life after a Heart Crisis*. 2010, New York: Penguin.

This book was written by a doctor, who had emergency heart surgery, and his wife, who was his caregiver. Both patient and caregiver will benefit from reading this book. The authors include very practical and useful advice, and will inspire you to get back to or start living a heart-healthy life.

Appendix

Before surgery considerations

1. How is the best way to prepare myself physically and emotionally for surgery?
2. Why should I have the surgery done at this hospital?
3. Can I set up a consultation appointment with my likely surgeon before making a decision?
4. Where should I go for a second opinion?
5. What pre-op testing will be done?
6. What changes in my medications will I need to make before surgery?
7. Will you accept my insurance as payment in full?
8. What accommodations are available for my family's stay on or near the hospital campus so that they can support me throughout the operation?

Surgery-specific questions

9. What symptoms make this surgery advisable?

10. What will likely happen if the operation is not done?
11. Will the operation improve my health and/or quality of life?
12. Are there any common complications after the operation?
13. Will I be able to listen to a CD during the operation? Can I have positive affirmations read to me before surgery?
14. How long does the surgery usually take?
15. What's the average length of hospital stay?
16. What is the progression of events after the operation?
17. How can I ensure that my surgeon will be doing the operation rather than senior residents? How many surgeons will be in the room?
18. What do you do for blood transfusions? Can family members donate? If I decide not to have blood products administered, does the hospital follow Bloodless Care Protocols?
19. For a valve surgery, what type of materials are you going to use (e.g. tissue, Gore-Tex, human) or will you use a mechanical valve?
20. What will you give for pain medication? How liberally?

21. When will family members be able to see me after surgery?

Hospital and Surgeon-specific concerns

22. How many surgeries for adults with my condition are done annually at this hospital and by whom?
23. What has been your success rate? Do you know about long-term success rates?
24. In what area does my surgeon specialize?
25. How many total heart surgery procedures are done at this hospital each year?
26. What is the overall mortality rate at this hospital?
27. What type of certification does the hospital and surgeon have? Board certified? Approved by the American Board of Specialties?

Post-op issues

28. What type of long-term follow-up does one need in the years after surgery (e.g., doctor visits, echocardiograms, EKGs, etc.)?
29. When will I be able to bathe and to wash my hair?

30. When will I be able to have my hair cut at a salon?
31. Are there any lifestyle restrictions post-surgery? Weight lifting, high-impact sports, or sports of any kind?
32. What is the normal recovery pattern?
33. What and how much support will I need during recovery?
34. What are my limitations during recovery?
35. What kinds of post-op medication might I be on (e.g. aspirin, blood thinner, blood pressure medications, etc.)? For life, or approximately how long?

9 781634 913829